Getting a Good Night's Sleep

How to fall asleep with only natural sleep remedies and
routines.

by Landon Sullivan

Table of Contents

What Causes Insomnia? Let's See What The Scientists Have to Say.

What do the smart guys, the sleep doctors and insomnia scientists have to say about getting a good night's sleep? Have they revealed any insights into why we cannot sleep? More importantly, do they have a blueprint for sound sleep, night after night?

First, let's take a look at insomnia and it's causes.
Insomnia - the inability to sleep soundly - can be caused by anything from stress and anxiety to growing older and even to changes that take place in your life.

While around 6% of the population has true, clinical insomnia with symptoms lasting over a month, at least 1 in 4 of us has occasional trouble sleeping soundly. I'm in the larger group that only has trouble sleeping occasionally.

One of my habits that leads to sleeplessness is drinking too many soda pops. It's been a lifelong weakness. I remember my Dad used to tease me when I was young. He'd occasionally call me, "Pepsi". (I'm glad that nickname didn't stick!)

I like to relax in the evening with a soft drink or two. Well, combine that with a stimulating television show like "Shark Tank" or "Better Call Saul" and you have a formula for laying in bed wide awake come bedtime!

Fortunately, the cure for my self imposed restlessness was simple. Cut back on the Cokes and drink a glass of water while watching my shows.

Did you notice a couple of other impediments to a good night's sleep in my evening routine? Yep, watching television and drinking fluids after about eight o'clock in the afternoon.

One of the main causes of insomnia is stress.

In fact, stress is probably the number one cause. That's not surprising, is it?

Stress can cause your mind to race at night. It can make sleep - much less a good night's sleep - nearly impossible.

Sometimes traumatic life events, such as the death of a loved one or a divorce, can bring stress home. Even if you have never had trouble sleeping in the past life changing events can make quality sleep nearly impossible.

Anxiety and depression can make it difficult to get a good night of sleep.

Many times anxiety disorders can cause you to lose sleep. Worrying that you will not be able to sleep soundly can become a self fulfilling concern. It becomes a vicious cycle that keeps you awake night after night.

Sometimes depression can cause you to sleep too much. Other times depression just will not allow you to get the good quality sleep you need.

If you suffer from anxiety or depression, see a doctor. It is important. You could have a medical condition like social anxiety disorder or post traumatic stress. They can help.

Parkinson's, Alzheimer's, and many other medical conditions can also lead to insomnia.

Unfortunately, the suffering caused by a wide variety of medical conditions can cause you to lose sleep. And it is true that many medications can get in the way of sound sleep, too.

Having a medical condition, taking medicines, and not sleeping well is a difficult situation. If this sounds like you, don't delay. Have a serious discussion with your doctor soon.

Well, what about coffee, cigarettes, and booze?

This just in: they are all bad for you. And, none of them really help you sleep soundly.

Yeah, I know. I slept pretty soundly after chugging a few beers back in my college days. We've all been there. Mostly.

But, truth be told I wasn't getting the sound, good quality sleep my tee-totaling roommate was. Come to think of it, I probably disturbed his sleep too.

Caffeine is a stimulant. The nicotine in tobacco is a stimulant as well. Smoking or having a cup of coffee in the evening can still be affecting you at bedtime.

Alcohol is a sedative and it can help you fall asleep. The trouble is that you will not sleep well. Booze can cause you to wake up in the middle of the night. It prevents you from entering the deep stages of sleep. Waking up in the middle of the night and not being able to get back to sleep because of a hangover is not a good feeling!

Poor eating and drinking habits - especially late in the day are not helpful.

A good diet plays a big part in a good night's sleep. What you eat and when you eat is important.

A large meal too close to bedtime can make it problematic to get to sleep. For one thing a full stomach can be uncomfortable. You will just toss and turn and have trouble settling down.

And if you get heartburn or indigestion that's not going to lead to pleasant dreams.

Drinking too much - even water - can cause you to have to wake up and use the bathroom in the middle of the night. Then you might have trouble getting back to sleep. try to cut off all fluids by about 3 hours before bedtime.

It's okay to have a light snack before going to bed. Something like a half turkey sandwich will settle the hunger pangs and help you sleep.

Irregular schedules mess up your body's rhythms.

Shift work can wreck your sleep patterns. Going from day to swing to graveyard shifts can really mess up the natural circadian rhythms of your body. These natural rhythms are like an internal timepiece. They regulate our sleep cycles among other things.

Our bodies like consistent routines, it seems. Maybe you have no control over your work schedule but it is easy to get out of sync during your off hours also.

It is best to have a consistent bedtime and wake up time 7 days a week. You may be tempted to stay up late on weekends but it's not a good idea. Staying up late on the weekends can send a ripple through our schedules and disrupt sound sleep patterns.

Try to keep to a routine. Early to bed and early to rise, while a tad boring - is probably best.

Your bedroom should only be used for two things. Care to guess?

Sleep and sex. So maybe a regular bedtime routine is not so boring, after all!

The mistake many of us - including John Lennon and Yoko Ono - make is to use the bedroom for things other than making love and sleeping soundly.

John and Yoko famously staged a bed-in for peace back in the 1960's. You and I may try and do a little paperwork, read a book, or watch television from our beds.

It's a mistake. You want to reserve your bedroom as a special place. Lounging around in bed all day will make it harder for you to get to sleep later on.

The bedroom environment needs to be just right.
I think of it as a Goldilocks Zone. the temperature needs to be just right. "Not too hot. Not too cold."

And a dark bedroom is best. Try to remove all sources of light including the glow of an alarm clock, a computer screen, or anything else.

You might want to check into blackout shades or even a sleep mask. Lights will keep you up.

Exercise can be good or bad when it comes to sleeping well.

It stands to reason that if you exercise too strenuously just before bedtime that you'll stay charged up and not be able to relax and doze off.

On the other hand, moderate, relaxing exercise can chase away the stress of the day and help you to sleep well.

It's much the same with taking a bath. A piping hot bath just before bedtime is probably not wise. On the other hand, a warm, relaxing bath with the lights down low can be a really good sleeping pill. Just unwind and release your troubles down the drain.

Getting older can cause insomnia, huh? Well, yes and no.

It's not so much that getting older causes insomnia. It's just that we oldsters tend to do some things that promote insomnia. So, yes there is a higher instance of not being able to get a good night of sleep among the older set.

As we get older we tend to become less active. We tend to take more pills. To be sure, there are age related reasons that we have insomnia more as we age. However, some factors are within our control.

It's hard to generalize because some insomnia in seniors is caused by changes in health. Some is caused by improper habits.

As you can see there are many things that can stand in the way of sleeping soundly.

Being unable to sleep can be from something as simple a having eaten a spicy meal late at night or it can stem from something more serious.

If you have trouble sleeping well night after night you should consult with the medical people. If there is any doubt, check it out.

For most of us who cannot get to sleep from time to time or who do not get a sound, restful night of sleep there are some simple, do-it-yourself fixes.

The fix may be correcting a bad soft drink habit like I did. Once I cut my sodas down and then out, I began to sleep much more soundly.

A lot of insomnia can be left outside the bedroom by a change in a person's outlook.

Once Harry Truman was asked how well he slept with all the troubles resting on his shoulders. Truman became President following the death of Franklin Roosevelt.

Not only did the burden of Commander-in-Chief become his, but it was Harry who had to make the ultimate decision of whether or not to drop "The Bomb."

Such awesome responsibilities would likely cause any of us to roam the White House hall until the wee hours of the morning.

But Harry told the reporter that he slept just fine. He explained that during the day he did the very best he could and since he had done his best, there was no need to worry about things any further.

President Truman's momentous decisions are still hotly debated to this day, but he was able to leave them at the bedroom door and sleep soundly through the night.

You and I can learn a lesson from this man from Independence, Missouri.

How Your Daily Routine Can Help You Sleep Soundly

I like to say that a good night's sleep begins the moment you wake up. I strongly believe that what you do throughout the day has an impact on the following night's rest.

You cannot expect to eat processed fast food and guzzle soda pop all day and sleep like a baby, now can you?

We can learn a lot from the folks that have gone before us. Sure, they didn't have all of our modern conveniences. But they lead simple lives in touch with nature. And they slept better too, I imagine. Good night, John Boy.

In trying to simplify my life (and sleep more soundly) I have developed a number of best practices. They work for me. I would encourage you to develop your own lists of sleep supporting habits. Experiment and see what does the trick for you.

Here are the things I strive to do from sun up to sundown in order to get great sleep night after night. Feel free to adopt and adapt as you see fit.

Early to rise.

I get up early, usually around 5 a.m to 5:30 a.m. There are so many advantages to rising early and it is especially helpful when establishing a good sleep routine.

Since I get up early and rarely take a nap, I'm very ready to hit the hay when bedtime rolls around. Waking up early and going to bed early are more in tune with the way nature intended for us to function.

I guess back on the farm in years gone by, everyone pretty much rose with the sun and went to bed shortly after sunset. Now we have the ability to stay up late and text on our smartphones, watch television, and do other stimulating things. We've conquered the night but perhaps not in a way that helps us sleep well.

Soon after I get up I drink a couple of glasses of water. I don't guzzle them down. It may take me an hour or an hour and a half but I find drinking those glasses of water gives me a calm energy and makes me more mentally alert.

Meet my personal trainer, Stretchy the Wonder Dog.

Sometimes I get up a little late. Sometimes I don't drink my water. But I never forget my morning walk.

As you probably guessed, that's because my dog, Stretchy, is always ready to go out and meet the world. She's part Jack Russell terrier, smarter than me, and knows how to get her way. We pretty much walk wherever she wants.

I really shouldn't complain. After all, I'm getting fresh air, exercise, and sunshine. Those are all good things that help to reduce stress and keep me healthy. They also help me sleep well at night.

Sunlight.

The circadian rhythm that governs our body's sleep cycle is controlled largely by light and dark. We need to get out in the sun during the day and we need it dark at night.

It's hard not to do almost the opposite in today's world. We can work indoors and hardly even see sunlight. And we can spend our evening hours in brightly lit rooms.

If you can, make it a point to get at least 2 hours of sunshine each day. Maybe you can take a walk during a lunch break. Perhaps you can go to a nearby park or walk in your neighborhood. Find a way. It's important.

During the workday.

When I was younger, I worked in construction. Falling asleep was not problem back then. As it says in Ecclesiastes, *"The sleep of a laboring man is sweet..."*

But now I'm older and have much more sedentary workdays. I tap, tap, tap, away at the computer. I don't think Solomon had much encouraging news to report about that!

But there are simple things I do to keep the stress from building up. I take breaks, do a little stretching or even a yoga pose or two.

While I might have a cup of coffee or so, I try not to overdo things.

Naps?

Naps are great. But napping too long can keep you awake at night. I seldom nap and never more than a half hour or so. And when I nap, it's not in my bedroom. Remember to reserve the bedroom for those two special activities!

In the evenings there are a few things I watch

Sometimes after a good dinner, I'm really ready to doze. I am a morning person and not really a ball of fire in the evenings.

But I resist the urge to nap after dinner. Maybe I'll take Stretchy for a short walk or maybe I'll do some chores around the house. I want to stay awake so that I'll be ready for some sound sleep come bedtime.

Another good strategy is to stop drinking fluids at least a couple of hours before bedtime. That way you are less likely to have to use the bathroom during the night.

From about 8 p.m. on, I'll have the house pretty dark. I may watch some television but I try and have a little break between my shows and going to sleep.

A nice, warm bath is a good way for me to unwind. It's ideal about an hour before you go to bed. A little reading also helps me to relax.

Bedtime!
Sometimes I just doze off. But when I need a little help getting to sleep, I have a couple of techniques that I use.

The first one is a really simple breathing exercise. I first learned of deep diaphragmatic breathing from a Tony Robbins book. He wrote that breathing deeply had many benefits.

Tony's method was a tad complicated. I simplified the method for my own needs. All I do is breath in deeply to a slow count of three. One...two...three. Then I naturally breath out and repeat.

Sometimes after about ten breaths or so, I lose track and am well on my way to sleep.

The second technique I sometimes use is to think about something good I did during the day.

If you think about it, even on your worst days, there is something good and worthwhile that you did.

It may be something small. Sometimes I think, "Well, I did walk my dog!" The important thing is to let your mind dwell on a positive.

The beauty of this method is that it keeps you from thinking about what your going to do tomorrow or what you messed up today. I believe it promotes more pleasant dreams. (It also motivates you to do something you can be proud of tomorrow!)

I get about seven hours of good sleep.
Since I usually go to bed around 10:30 at night, I only get around 7 hours of sleep. That is all I require. I think 8 hours would just be too much for me.

Everyone is different. We all have need differing amounts of sleep. You probably know already just how much nightly sleep best suits you.

If not, experiment. you'll quickly discover the right amount of nightly sleep that suits you.

Find the routine that works best for you.

I given you an outline of the daily routine that supports me. This is what I try and follow each day to sleep soundly night after night. You are welcome to give it a try.

Probably a better approach would be for you to examine your current daily patterns to spot areas that could use an improvement. You might want to keep a journal for about a week.

In the journal you could keep track of when you get up and when you go to sleep. You could note how well you slept.

You could track meals, exercise sessions, how much time you were out in the sunshine and fresh air. You can make your journal as extensive or as simple as you want. Over a week, it can reveal some interesting habits and patterns.

When you make changes, I think it's best to give them time. Give them a fair chance. You body need a little while to adjust. When I realized I was drinking all that soda in the evenings, I took some time to reduce the amount and to taper off gradually.

If I would have tried to quit cold turkey, I probably would have had even more trouble getting to sleep. I would have given up and failed. Instead of cutting off the soft drinks all at once, I simply reduced the amount slowly. If I still craved a drink, I took a sip.

It's also a good idea to replace a bad habit with a good habit. As I tapered of those bad old soft drinks I replaced them with ice water.

Stacking habits gives the best results.

For most of us, a change or two can have a big impact on the quality of our sleep. Establish a normal, consistent routine. Create a good environment in the bedroom.

I think it is a good idea to implement one strategy at a time. That way you can be sure if it works for you. Gradually over time you can add more habits to your daily routine. There is true power in stacking good habits throughout your day.

Seeking professional help.

We can do a lot to help ourselves sleep better in most cases. But there are times when the problem is more serious. If you have any concern at all, it is best to talk with your doctor. Your doctor may reassure you or find something that needs to be taken care of.

The lack of sleep can be a serious, even life threatening condition at times. Don't guess. Don't put it off. Do the best thing for you and your health.

Stress and the Loss of Sleep.

Are you under a lot of stress? Have you recently gone through a traumatic experience? Is your job getting the best of you?

If you are like most of us, you likely said "Yes" to one of these questions or similar questions about stress. It's well established that we live in a high stress culture.

Many times the stresses of the day contribute to bouts of insomnia at night. Stress can make it both difficult for us to fall asleep and can affect the quality of the sleep we do get. So if we can get rid of the stress, we can sleep more soundly.

What exactly is stress?

We all know what stress is. We've all felt it. Stress can be defined as *an emotional or mental strain resulting from demanding circumstances.*

Stress can be caused by external circumstances. Imagine a brand new firefighter hearing the alarm go off at the station house for the very first time. That would have to produce a certain amount of stress.

Internal circumstances can cause stress as well. Worrying about that job interview or your next sales call can cause stress. Thinking about the meal you need to prepare for the in-laws can do the trick. And our rookie firefighter can lay awake worrying about the fire alarm sounding.

Stress comes in many forms but how can we get rid of it?

We have already discussed the importance of having a good daily routine. Having a set bedtime and wake up time is a good foundation for getting a good night's sleep. A winding down time before bedtime is also a good, supportive habit to develop. It helps us get rid of accumulated stresses before we go to bed.

Next, we need to identify the causes of our stress. Sometimes we can eliminate a cause. Let's say your favorite television show comes on just before bedtime. You get really caught up in the action and take the show to bed with you.

That's stress and it keeps you from going right to sleep. I know it's hard to stop watching your favorites shows. But maybe you can still watch it - just not right before bedtime.

Maybe you can record your show and watch it a couple of hours before your go to sleep. I sometimes get caught up in watching baseball games and regret it later! Extra innings, oh no! (Solution: Sports Center in the morning!)

In instances such as these we can reduce stress simply by making it a priority to do so. But other stressful situations are not as simple to solve. Some are almost out of our control entirely.

External stress throughout the day.

While we try to fill our days with happy and rewarding events, the real world encroaches into this fantasy.

Daily stress may begin building up on your morning commute to work. It can even start before you leave the house. Making sure everyone is awake, cleaned and dressed, and fed breakfast can move the stress meter up.

Office politics, deadlines, interruptions. The list of things that can cause stress is voluminous.

Even though external stress is beyond our control, there is something we can do.

By definition, external events that cause stress are beyond our control. What is within our control is how we interpret those events and how we respond to them.

For example, one day years ago I was out walking. I used to go on fairly long walks back then. I'd gotten about to my turn around point and was feeling pretty good.

Then all of a sudden, a car full of high school guys buzzes past. The driver lays on the horn and one of the hooligans yell something at me.

As they sped down the road my adrenaline shot up. My heart was pounding and I was mad! I kept replaying the scene over and over in my mind. "You jerks", I thought. "What a bunch of cowards! Wait 'til I catch up with you!"

But then I caught myself. I realized what I was doing to me. I mean who really cares about a bunch of kids out joyriding?

So I played a little mind game on the way home. Since I'd really not heard what the young man said I decided to pretend that he was yelling an encouraging message to me.

"Way to go! Keep up the good work!"

It was all pretty silly but it helped me calm down and enjoy the rest of my walk. I could have stewed all night about that little incident. Thankfully, I was able to take control of my mind and not let an insignificant incident fester.

The point is: we have the choice in how to represent things in our mind. We can consciously interpret events in ways that benefit and empower us. I didn't give away that power to those kids. Don't you give your power away to others.

Sometimes things are more serious.

Okay, I'll grant you that not letting those kids ruin my walk just took a little maturity. But what about when the external cause of stress is much more serious?

What about when your job, your marriage, or even your life is on the line? It's hard to look at those stresses in a positive light, right?

Right. There are situation in life when it is difficult - even impossible - to cast things is a warm fuzzy feeling. It's good to develop the skill to look at things in a positive light as much as possible.

But tragic and catastrophic things happen. Some things you just have to suffer through.

How do you manage stress when your world is seemingly coming apart?

There's no easy answer here. I lost plenty of sleep when my Mom passed away. We were very close and I was here primary caregiver for years. Our lives basically revolved around each other. Now she was gone.

During the dark days after her passing, I visited a friend. I had not spent time with Eddie in a while. What I found was shocking.

Eddie had been through some tough times, too. He tried to comfort me and give me some encouragement. But all I could hear in him was the drugged up rambling of someone still playing the victim.

It open my eyes. I was not going to seek relief in pills or booze. I was determine not to play the pathetic victim. I would face the situation head on. I would live a life that would make my Mom proud.

That's really the shortest and easiest road back. Face the facts and take the pain. There's no easy way to start reclaiming the quality of your life.

It's been less than two months since Mom passed away but I'm sleeping pretty good. I still have to give myself a talking to on occasion. But I'm sure glad I didn't turn to any short term crutch like medication.

Sometimes medication may be the best way to reduce stress and get some sleep.

I realize medications prescribed by your physician can at times be the best way for you to deal with your stresses. Just be careful. I've seen people hooked on their pills. I am sure you have, too.

What are some natural ways to reduce or get rid of stress?

Take a deep breath or several.

One of the quickest ways I know of the get rid of stress is through breathing deeply from your diaphragm. There are many different deep breathing techniques but I prefer to keep it simple.

I just breathe in for a count or 3 or 4 and then breath out naturally. The key is to let your diaphragm rise and fall pulling air deep into your lungs. After several good breaths, I can really tell a difference in my stress levels.

Try this method or other similar breathing methods like yogic breathing. Imagine breathing deeply through one nostril and slowly out through the other. You don't actually breath through a single nostril but trying to take your mind off of those other stressful things.

I take a minute or two several times during the day to relax with deep breathing. It's especially effective just before bedtime. And if you wake up during the night, a few slow deep breaths might just put you back into a sound slumber.

An exercise session can really knock out that stress.

Whether it's a brisk walk in the outdoors or an energetic workout with your favorite fitness guru, exercise can tame the stress monster.

In addition to getting the blood circulating and the breathing going, you can get lost in many forms of exercise.

When I'm really stressed out I'll pop in a workout video and try to really apply myself and just get into the session. A grueling yoga workout can sometimes transform me. Oooom.

Runners know all about the so called runner's high. This is when the body releases endorphins into the body. This natural chemical promotes a positive feeling within the body. Other forms of exercise also release endorphins.

Live on the sunny side of the street.

As mentioned earlier our attitude has a large impact on how we deal with stress. Have you noticed that a large percentage of elderly people live with an attitude of gratitude.

Do you think we become more grateful as we age? Or, do you suppose naturally grateful folks live longer?

Eat or drink something.

When we are stressed just about any food is comforting. But some foods are way better than others. Berries and nuts tend to rank high as a stress relieving snack.

Chamomile tea is very soothing. It's a great drink to help you unwind in the evening.

In moderation, chocolate can improve your mood and help you get over a stress filled day. Dark chocolate is best.

Oatmeal is great. It fights stress by causing your brain to produce the feel good chemical serotonin. Start your day off with a bowl of steel cut oatmeal and maybe you will have a stress free day!

Eat foods rich in Vitamin B. I mentioned nuts earlier. Beans, eggs, peas, and meat products have lots of this stress relieving vitamin.

Drink a good amount of water regularly. Develop a habit of drinking water throughout each day. I think you will be impressed at the health benefits of water.

The best stress reducer of all? A good night's sleep!

If you've been having trouble sleeping soundly due to stress, I believe that by developing good habits the quality of your night's rest will improve.

Begin to stack one sleep enhancing habit on top of another and you'll be pleasantly amazed at the difference it makes. Sleeping well will enable you to better handle the stress that comes your way each day.

With less stress build up and better ways to relieve it, you change the vicious cycle of stress and bad sleep to a virtuous cycle of good sleep and lower stress.

It only takes some effort and commitment to change bad habits and develop good habits. I think you will find the reward of sound sleep is well worth the effort.

The Dangers of a Lack of Sleep.

The lack of sleep can have many consequences. Some are very serious. Lack of sleep can even lead to death.

Lack of sleep can lead to accidents.

Being drowsy behind the wheel of a car can be dangerous for you and the other people on the road. Reaction times can be slowed to about the same degree as driving drunk.

Workplace accidents are more likely to happen when you are suffering from a lack of sleep. Likewise, home accidents are more frequent for those that are sleep deprived. Sleepiness makes you more likely to suffer an accident.

You could become more at risk for serious health conditions.

Chronic sleep loss can put you at risk for medical conditions ranging from heart trouble to diabetes.

If you suffer from insomnia you are more likely to have a heart attack or stroke. A single night without adequate sleep can cause your blood pressure to be elevated throughout the day if you already suffer from hypertension.

You are more likely to gain weight if you do not get the sleep you need.

Cortisol, the stress hormone, is increased in your body when you fail to get enough sleep. The hormone that tells you when you've eaten enough, Leptin, is lowered.

The appetite stimulant, Ghrelin, is increased. Higher levels of insulin are also released.

Lack of sleep creates the perfect storm for giving you the munchies and storing more fat.

Your brain activity becomes impaired.
The brain needs sleep. Lack of sound sleep effects the brain in a number of ways.

Your memory, attention span, and the ability to perform simple tasks can suffer when you do not get adequate sleep. Tempers are more likely to flare and mood swings become more common. You can even become giddy - which is not so bad!

The exhausted brain sleeps and makes you sleepy and sluggish. If you deprive yourself of needed sleep, the brain will go into micro-sleep sessions.

These involuntary sleep periods can last for seconds or minutes. They can happen anywhere, including when you are driving. Many tragic accidents have happen due to the lack of sleep with planes, trains, and automobiles.

Trips and falls are more likely due to several effects of being in a sleepy state. Micro-sleep, lack of attention, and clumsiness can all trip you up.

The lack of sleep for teenagers.
Teens need a good amount of sleep each night. They typically need about 8 to 10 hours. Less than one in six get enough sleep.

It is not unusual for teens to have crazy sleep patterns. They are know to stay up late and sleep in on the weekends. Of course this irregular routine plays havoc with their internal body rhythms.

For a teenager the lack of sleep can affect their studies and even their social life.

Concentration and problem solving abilities are hurt. You might forget when that homework assignment is due or when General Washington crossed the Delaware.

Names and number become more difficult to remember. That can hurt both your Scholastic work and your social game.

The lack of sleep can make you moody. It can lead to antisocial behaviors such as yelling and otherwise being a jerk. That won't go over well with your friends or your instructors.

Lack of sleep can make it more likely you will develop acne or some other skin predicament. The tendency to eat the wrong things increases. Along with that your weight is more likely to increase.

Teens need to prioritize sleep in order to excel. They need a regular sleep routine both during the week and on weekends.

Teens need to turn off the computer, television, smartphone, tablet, and other devices in the period preceding bedtime. Calming activities such as reading, taking a bath, or relaxing outside will set the stage for a good night's sleep.

Parents play a huge role in establishing an optimal sleep routine. They need to set boundaries and discuss the importance of a good sleep routine with their youngsters. It helps if Mom and Dad set a good example.

When teenagers go away to college or move away from home, there will be many distractions and interruption to good sleep habits. Teens need to become aware of these and make the best adjustments possible. Good luck.

The lack of sleep when pregnant.

Most women have problems sleeping during pregnancy. This is to be expected. With so many changes happening, it is little surprise that pregnant women suffer from insomnia.

In addition to the emotional and physical change that happen during pregnancy, women also cite several other factors that make sound sleep difficult.

It is challenging to get comfortable in bed.
Sleeping on your left side is best while pregnant. But if you are not used to sleeping in this position it may initially feel uncomfortable. It may take some time to get used to sleeping in this position.

The added weight of pregnancy may cause you to ache all over. It may be harder to get comfortable with a large belly.

When you do get to sleep, a kick or two from the baby can wake you up.

You will need to go to the bathroom more often. Leg cramps are common. And you are anxious to deliver the newborn.

Insomnia is very common during pregnancy but usually not harmful to the baby. Just like a person who is not pregnant, the lack of sleep can put you a risk while driving as well as other situations where you need your full concentration.

Many of the same techniques useful while your not pregnant - have a sleep routine, unwind before bedtime, reduce stress - will help when you are with child.

In addition there are several other tactics you can use to encourage sleep. Make use of pillows to support your body. A knee pillow can help you be more comfortable on your left side.

Realize that it is normal to have trouble sleeping during pregnancy. Try not to worry. Worry only makes the problem worse.

Take advantage of exercise classes that are specially geared for pregnant women. Yoga and stretching classes can relieve you of stress. You will also be able to meet and socialize with other pregnant women. You can comfort and support one another.

Lack of sleep for the elderly.

It is normal for sleep patterns to change as we age. But sleeping soundly is crucial to the health of older people. The lack of sleep has been associated with dementia and cognitive impairment. You are more likely to fall if you have not had enough sleep.

Sleep disorders can cause an increase chance of death.

Diseases, such as Alzheimer's can change sleep patterns. Health issues that seniors have can make them more likely to develop insomnia, sleep apnea, or other sleep disorders.

There are many ways available to help the elderly sleep better.
If you are elderly, you are likely well acquainted with your primary physician. She or he should know your medical conditions well. You and your caregivers need to discuss your sleep difficulties and decide on a course of action.

In addition to any prescribed medications, it may be good for you to stay active and engaged during the day. Depending on your particular situation, you might benefit from getting out of the house - even for short trips to the grocery or hairdresser.

Sitting outside on a porch or deck can help you relax and sleep well at night. Socializing with friends and family is probably a better way to relax than watching reruns of "Matlock".

Staying out of bed during the day (as much as possible) and taking less naps can help some elderly folks sleep better at night.

Caregivers play an increasingly important role in the lives of seniors. They need to be concerned about helping the loved one under their care to sleep.

They also need to take care of themselves as well. An irritable, overtired caregiver can exacerbate the sleeping difficulties of the one they are trying to assist.

Lack of sleep for busy, Type A people.

This is a culture that almost glorifies a too busy to sleep lifestyle. I often hear people complain that they are just so busy that they "don't have time to sleep".

They almost wear their hectic lifestyle as a badge of honor. Well, kudos to them for hustling but the dangerous side effects of too little sleep can catch up to the overachiever as well.

In fact, the Type A person has a tendency to overlook and minimize the effects of sleep deprivation. The more deprived of sleep the person becomes, the less they are able to recognize they are in need of sleep.

Get a good night's rest. Take it seriously.

Don't think you are the one that can get by without any sleep. Don't be the one to kill someone else on the highway. Lack of sleep can impair you just like drinking.

I'm no saint. Once I drove for 40 hours straight in order to get home when on leave from the Navy. When I got on the final interstate highway just 50 miles from home, I took off in the wrong direction. I drove 20 to 30 miles before I even realize my mistake.

How foolish. I could have killed myself or some innocent person. Finally, I made it home.

What's the first thing I did? Hugged my Mom and went to bed!

Quality Time Before Bedtime.

The hours before you go to bed help set the stage for a good night's sleep. The routine we follow then largely determines how well we sleep at night.

If you do not currently have a before bedtime routine that supports a good night sleep, you need to change.

Change is hard and staying in your current routine is comfortable. You may know you need to change and develop good, supportive sleep habits but you're having a hard time making them stick.

So how do you change from a bad before bedtime routine to a good one?

I believe that the key to successfully making any change is to gain leverage over the situation. The change you are working toward needs to become very important to you.

You need to gain leverage over the situation. Then you'll be well motivated to take the action you need to take.

Find a big enough "Why".

The best way I have found to replace a bad habit with a good one is to focus on why you are making the change. If your reason why is important enough, you will be successful. You will make the change.

The "why" must be important to you. We have already looked at a number of reasons that sound sleep is important.

Getting a good night's sleep can affect your health, it can affect the quality of your relationships.

The lack of sleep can be dangerous. It can cause mental impairment. It can cause you to fall asleep - even when operating a motorized vehicle. The lack of sleep could even kill you.

These are all strong reasons for you to place a high priority on getting proper rest every night. But the only reasons that will compel you to make lasting changes are the one's that matter most to you.

Maybe for you the reason that gives you strong motivation is your family. Perhaps you realize that you have been testy and not present around your wife and kids.

You hate that and realize that resting well can transform your attitude into what you want it to be. You're ready and motivated to turn off the computer, cut short the sports program and get your mind in a good state for bedtime.

Maybe you realize that the lack of sleep is contributing to that jelly belly you are now toting around. Your eyes have been opened to the ways the lack of sleep causes you to gain weight. You despise the way you look. You feel uncomfortable in your clothes.

You are ready to change a few things and start getting a good night's rest. You know proper rest will be a good foundation for your weight shredding plans.

What is your "Why"?

I urge you to take a few minutes now and ask yourself, "What is my strong, compelling reason to make the changes needed to start sleeping well? What is my"Why"?

Those are powerful questions. Take your time and answer them well. They can give you the motivation to carry through and establish a great pre-sleep routine.

Here's the key.

I hope you will write your "why" down. Commit it to paper. Make it emotional. And, read it with emotion at least once a day.

It does not have to be long. You can change it. Here's a sample.

I, (your name), realize that I have been moody and very unpleasant to the people I love most,(name them). I realize that sleeping better at night will tend to make me a more pleasant individual. I am willing to make the necessary changes in my evening routine in order to sleep soundly at night.

I commit to taking the hour before I go to bed, 10:00 to 11:00 p.m. and sitting out on my back porch and unwinding with my wife and children in the cool, fresh air without any communication devices or other stresses.

Go ahead. Write your own. Make yours better than mine!

Now let's take a look at some of the things you need to include and exclude in the time before you go to bed.

Here's a list of some habits and practices you can adopt to help you get ready for bed. There is probably no need to do the whole list. But the first item is crucial.

Go to bed at the same time every night.

The routine of sticking to a bedtime - and also a wake up time - is central sleeping well almost every night.

Did you know your body has a master clock? True. The suprachiasmatic nucleus in the brain keeps all the body's clocks in sync.

Simply put, when you have a regular sleep schedule you are working with your body internal mechanisms instead of fighting against them.

If you have ever flown across several time zones, you know it takes your body some time to adjust to the new time. Or, maybe you are like me and have trouble adjusting your sleep schedule when the government moves the clocks backward and forward.

Establishing a routine is important when it comes to getting to sleep. That is one reason I suggest you keep your routine simple.

Don't try and run down a checklist each evening. You'll be creating stress instead of relieving it. Choose a couple of habits and follow them. Maybe add a single habit and go from there. Perhaps one good habit is all you'll ever need.

Eating and drinking wisely before bed can promote sound sleep.
It's a good idea to really limit liquids and food for a couple of hours before bedtime. I sometimes make a green drink with my juice machine and sip on it after dinner. The green vegetable juices really mellow me down. The effect reminds me of drinking a beer without the bad side effects.

Stimulants, like sodas and coffee, should be on your do not go there list. And while an alcoholic drink may relax you at first, they have a nasty habit of waking folks up in the middle of the night. So stay away from the alcohol, too.

If you do need a snack before bedtime, try something light. A half turkey sandwich is what I always recommend.

Exercise can help you sleep - or keep you awake.
I find that yoga or stretching exercises help me to unwind. Each of these workout types promote deep breathing and relaxation. A short walk at dusk with my dog also helps me wind down.

High intensity exercises too close to bedtime can energize you and make sleep close to impossible. Lifting heavy weights or high intensity interval training is best done in the morning.

Turn the lights down low or go outside.
A few minutes out on the deck will sometimes calm me down when nothing else seems to do the trick. I use unwinding on the outside deck as a cheat when I've watched a ballgame late into the night. Perhaps as little as 15 minutes will put me in a state where I'm ready to fall asleep.

Turning the lights down inside is also conducive to getting your body ready for sleep. Light and dark play an important role the chemical processes of our system. Try to get out in the sunlight during the day. Even if you work indoors, take breaks whenever you can.

Then when the sun goes down, lower the lighting and create an environment that will help you get ready for sleepy time.

A warm bath can relax you.
Taking a warm - but not hot - bath is a good way to relax in the evenings. It is a good idea. Just don't take a bath right before you go to bed. Try to get your bath at least 30 minutes before you go to bed.

Meditation or prayer.
Spend a few minute of quiet, quality time either with yourself or a higher being. Look at the big picture and realize what is important and what is just noise.

Listen to calming music or the birds singing outside.
The birds in the trees, the chirping of crickets, or a wonderful song can take you away from your everyday stresses and put you in the mood to sleep well.

Listen to a favorite mellow song and quietly sing along. Music can take you to a different state of mind.

Stop and smell the roses.
Aromas can help with stress and anxiety. That's the idea behind aromatherapy.

You can literally sniff fresh flowers or smell essential oils such a lavender. Some people say the smell of coffee helps them relax. Some find the aroma of citrus fruits helps them relax.

Unwind with good friends.
Now these friends can be human or the four legged type of friends. Me and my buddy Stretchy like to spend a little quality time before beddy - bye.

With your human friend, a relaxed conversation and some good laughs can let the pressures of your day slip away.

Develop a before bedtime routine that works for you.

It's all about what does the job for you. Maybe you will develop one key habit or ritual that leaves you ready for bed. Maybe you can mix things up and have several relaxation strategies in your arsenal. It's up to you.

Any before bed relaxing works best in combination with a day that is low stress.

It's easier to relax in the evening if your day hasn't been spent building up stress. If you can lower the workday aggravations or at least release some stress during the day, your evenings will be instantly calmer.

I know it's easier said than done. But the entire day from when you wake up until you lay down your head influences how well you sleep and how easily you doze off.

And just as your daytime hours set the stage for the evening hours before bedtime, a quality time before bedtime ultimately sets the stage for going to bed.

Create a Great Bedroom Environment for a Good Night's Sleep.

Your whole day leading up to bedtime can make it easy or difficult to sleep soundly. That is true. But one of the biggest factors in sleeping well night after night is your bedroom environment.

You can establish a sleep routine, eat right, manage stress, and unwind before bed, and still toss and turn all night. If your bedroom is not a good sleeping place, your chances of sleeping well are crushed.

It's true that if you are sleepy enough, you can sleep just about anywhere. For years, I slept on board a Navy ship in overcrowded and miserable conditions. From the stories I've heard, my Army and Marine comrades had much worse sleeping conditions.

But while you can sleep in a rack, on a boat, or in a foxhole, who wants that? We all want a bedroom that helps us go to sleep and sleep wonderfully. There is nothing quite like that feeling of being well rested when you first wake up.

Taking inventory of your bedroom.

Is your bedroom currently a wonderful refuge that invites you to slumber land? Are there things you would like to change? Does your bedroom need a makeover? Will a few simple adjustments help? Let's take a look.

The distractions.

A golden rule for the bedroom is that it should be used for two things only. It should only be a sanctuary for sleep and sex. It should not be a television room. It should not double as an office. It's not a place for computers or any other electronic devices.

If you are using your bedroom for more than it's intended uses, stop it. If at all possible, take out the office desk that's squeezed in there. Make an honest effort. Put the television somewhere else. Get the devices out of there.

This is your bedroom; your sanctuary. Develop the mindset that your bedroom is the place you get away to. Make it the room you reward yourself with after a long day. Make it special.

The bed.

If you are having a problem sleeping it could be your bed that's causing you to not sleep well. A good bed along with a good mattress and high quality bedding work together to support sound sleep.

Let's start with the bed itself. Is it large enough? Is there ample space for you and your partner? Is it in good shape or is it old and starting to breakdown?

If you are not answering "Yes" to these questions, it may be time to get a new bed. Beds are a pricey investment but a new bed may be well worth the price tag if it improves the quality of your sleep.

Maybe it's the mattress that's causing you grief. Is it too firm or too soft? Maybe it is just too old. The experts recommend we replace mattresses about every 8 years.

Maybe all you need to transform your bed into a sleep haven are good quality bedding materials. They can make all the difference. Pillows and sheets and blankets are so important we'll look at each topic individually.

The pillows.

The purpose of a bed pillow is the support a person's head. By keeping your head elevated and your neck in a good neutral alignment, the pillow can have a considerable effect in the quality of sleep you receive.

Different pillows work better for different styles of sleep. For instance, a person that sleeps on their side would enjoy a thicker pillow more than a person who sleeps on their back. That is just because sleeping on your side elevates the head and neck further away from the mattress than does sleeping on your back.

The idea is to keep the head, neck, and spine in alignment. Anyone that has awakened with a headache or a neck hurting can attest to the importance of sleeping with a good pillow.

There are many types of pillows from which you can choose. I remember the old goose down pillows from my childhood. They were suppose to give you such a good night's sleep.

You can still find them and many folks still say they are the best. I think it just a nostalgic choice, myself. But a good old goose down pillow may be just right for you.

I prefer a good memory foam pillow. I sleep some on my back and some on my sides at night. a good thicker memory foam pillow works best for me.

Other pillow choices you may want to look into include buckwheat, polyester fiberfill, organic wool or cotton pillows.

Even a good pillow can just get old. You should consider replacing pillows every two years or so. Not only can they wear out but they can also accumulate bed bugs and other particles that can cause allergic reactions. That in turn can cause a rotten night's sleep.

New pillows can make a huge difference. Put some thought into your purchase and be willing to invest in quality.

Pillows 2.0

In addition to traditional pillows, there is now a growing array of specialty pillows. These are sometimes referred to as positioners.

Maternity or pregnancy pillows are very popular. They are large pillows that support the whole body. Several different designs (J -shaped, C-shaped, U-shaped, etc.) are on the market. Women say these support pillows help them sleep comfortably even when they are not pregnant.

Foam wedges, horseshoe shaped neck pillows, knee pillows, and even total body pillows are made to support and position you for a more comfortable sleep.

While some of these seem a bit gimmicky, you may find one that helps you sleep. That's all that counts, after all.

The sheets and blankets.

I bet you already knew that natural fabrics like Egyptian cotton are more comfortable than synthetic fibers. It just makes sense. Synthetic fibers are more likely to trap in heat. Good quality cotton sheets breathe and let air circulate better.

Higher thread count sheets are more comfortable - to a point. 400 is the magic number when it comes to thread count. Those higher thread counts use synthetic finishes and probably are just weaving two textiles together.

Clean sheets make a difference when it comes to sleeping well. You should wash sheets about once a week. The detergent you use needs to be considered here. Your sensitive skin could be affected by a harsh detergent so use a mild detergent and rinse the sheets thoroughly.

In the summer or just when you are more active, it's a good idea to change sheets more often. Also factor in whether or not you clean up before bedtime.

You should also wash new sheets a couple of times before putting them into service. Packaging materials may contain ingredients that would interfere with your sleep. You want to wash that stuff away.

Bedding does not last forever. If your sheets and blankets are worn out, it may be time to replace them. A fresh set every couple of years is about right. Fresh sheets, pillowcases and blankets feel better and more fresh. Changing the way your bed feels can make a big difference in the quality of your sleep.

The temperature.

A cool bedroom is ideal for restful sleep. A very cool temperature between 60 and 68 degrees is ideal. Bedroom temperatures above 75 degrees and below 54 thwart sleep.

Four hours or so after you drift off to sleep, your core temperature is at it's lowest point. A cooler bedroom mimics the body's natural drop in temperature. Scientist think this is why the cool room helps with sleeping.

But there is a problem with a cool bedroom...

Maybe while reading this you've thought, *"Yes, but my hands and feet freeze when the temperature is that cold!"*

Well, you are correct! While a cool bedroom is great news in general, cold hands and feet are not going to help you get to sleep.

You need to keep your hands and feet warm while keeping the bedroom cool. Warm socks and mittens - or even a hot water bottle - are fixes to this dilemma.

The darkness.

Sleeping at night in a bedroom that is completely, totally dark helps us sleep soundly and promotes better overall health. It is natural for humans to sleep in the dark of night. We are programmed to do so.

Bedrooms today are not just a room with a bed. We cram them with lighting, digital clocks, televisions, and all sorts of electronic devices.

Even the light of a Kindle reader or a smartphone screen has enough light to disrupt sleep. Blue light disrupts the body's production of melatonin.

The bedroom needs to be very dark when we are sleeping.

Take an inventory of your bedroom.

If you are having trouble sleeping soundly a few easy changes could solve your problem. The odds are good that you need to make some changes in order to get a better night's sleep.

The televisions, digital clocks, and computer devices all need to move. Anything that have a glowing screen or even a red light is out. The nightlight is no longer an option. Make the room as dark as possible.

If there is any light coming in from a window, block it out with blackout curtains. Make the room as dark as you safely can.

If you need some light for safety, that is fine. Make exceptions for safety but otherwise, the darker the better.

The noise level.

Noise can keep you up at night. Even the tick tock, tick tock of a clock or watch can be enough sometimes.

Noises can come from outside the bedroom. Dogs bark, cars rumble, and neighbors can be loud.

Sometimes the noises coming from the bedroom can be even worse. A snoring bed mate can have you sleeping on the couch - or vice versa. If you still have that television or computer in the bedroom, those noisemakers can keep you awake.

Eliminate all the noises you can and try to mask or muffle those sounds you cannot stop. Sometimes you can easily block a noise. It can be as easy as closing a window or door.

I can't hear or be disturbed by the ticking clock in the bathroom across the hall when the bathroom door is shut. But if I forget to shut that door it will sometimes keep me awake. Look around and see what noise makers you can easily take care of.

Sometimes it helps if you can muffle sounds that might otherwise wake you. White noise machines emit a calm sound that resembles a rain storm or gentle waves.

These gentle sound can distract you from your worries and mask other sleep disturbing sounds. You can invest in one of these or even listen to one via YouTube (if you still haven't removed that computer!).

A snoring bed mate is one of the toughest noise problems to solve. One strategy you might try is to get to sleep before your roomie. Earplugs are another way to go. Separate bedrooms are another option.

But really the snoring needs to be looked into. Snoring can be a dangerous thing. It's possible your partner has a medical condition that needs medical attention. Perhaps the snoring stems from a correctable habit such as drinking alcohol in the evenings.

Snoring is more than just irritating noise that keeps you awake. It's something that needs to be fixed.

The smells.

Do not overlook the role pleasant smells play in enhancing your sleep environment. A clean, fresh smelling bedroom is inviting.

Certain aromas can have a more specific effect on your sleep. The evidence is indicating that lavender may lower blood pressure and heart rate.

Clean bedding that is washed in a pleasing smelling detergent can help most folks sleep more comfortably. So keep your sheets clean and place a drop of lavender scented oil on your pillow.

The bedroom. Your night time sanctuary.

Once you adopt the mindset that your bedroom is a special retreat and not some catch all room, you can reap the rewards to sound sleep almost each and every night.

It becomes a place your treat with care and respect. I look forward to laying my head down each night in a bedroom that is solely and specifically a place to rest at night.

No longer do I read a book in bed. Nor do I wallow around while watching a favorite television show. I make my bed when I wake up and it's ready for me at bedtime. I keep my bedding fresh and clean. I keep the bedroom cool, dark, clean and fresh smelling.

The blackout shade is pulled and all the lights and noise makers are somewhere else.

It took some effort and costs to transform my night time environment. But I have been repaid many times over in the quality sleep I get night after night.

Now I Lay Me Down to Sleep...

Bedtime! Your reward for a day well spent. You woke up right on time. You got some sunlight and managed the stresses of the day really well. You spent a relaxing evening and unplugged from the devices well before bedtime. You exercised a little and took a warm relaxing bath about a half hour before the appointed hour.

The temperature is nice and cool. The bedroom is nice and dark. The sheets are clean and fresh with just a touch of lavender oil providing a pleasing aroma.

You hit the sack and there's just one problem. You cannot get to sleep!

Don't panic. The good news is that if you've followed a sleep supporting routine, you'll drift right off into slumber most nights. But there are nights when - despite your best efforts - sleep does not come easily.

Fortunately, there are several effective ways you can help yourself get into a sound sleep. You just need to find out why you are having trouble getting to sleep.

Maybe you are thinking about what you need to do tomorrow. Perhaps you are worried about something you left undone today.

Are you excites, sad, or angry? Are you in pain?

Maybe you have gotten so much good rest lately that you are just not sleepy at all!

Once you know why you are restless, you can take the most effective steps.

Do stop thinking about tomorrow.

One of the most common things keeping us awake is a racing mind. We lay our heads down on the pillow and our brains just keep whizzing away.

I have a tendency to worry about tomorrow. I find myself making plans and worrying about what I'm going to say and do. Maybe you tend to focus on mistakes you made during the past day.

Each of these patterns is almost guaranteed to make sleep more difficult. Even if you do fall asleep you are likely to be restless.

Instead of regretting past mistakes or being anxious about the future, a good practice is to pick out something you did well in the past day and go to sleep focused to that. I often do this and it helps me to go to sleep and to sleep soundly.

When you think of it, there is always *something* good you did each day. It does not need to be earth shaking. It can be a small thing like walking your dog. It just needs to be something positive that you can focus on and leave the worries and anxiety behind.

For example, let's say you are the star shortstop in a big baseball playoff. Today you struck out all 3 times you came to bat. You booted a double play ball hit right to you.

You ripped your pants falling down the steps of the dugout. You are sore, hurting, and mad! There's another big game tomorrow but you are in no mood to sleep soundly.

Okay, stop the script running through your head.

As you lay down to sleep, the past days miseries keep running through your mind. You are making each miscue larger and more vivid as time goes by. Then you start worrying about the big game tomorrow. That starting pitcher is tough. How can you ever get a hit off of him?

The clock is ticking. You are not getting any sleep. But then you stop and remember a sleep technique you have been practicing.

At first you feel foolish but you give it a try. You remember something good you did today. You took the rookie left fielder under your wing. You spent some time with him and encouraged him. You could see him relax. He played pretty well.

Now your mind starts to relax. You focus on this single positive in a day full of negatives. When your mind wanders back to the unpleasant things you guide it back to this good moment.

Soon you fall asleep and rest well. The next day you hit the game winning home run and your team goes on to win the playoff. Because you gained control of your thoughts and had a sound sleep, you were able to perform at your best.

You may not be the shortstop.

True, you may not really be the star shortstop. But you do need to perform at your best each day. Whether you are a homemaker, whether you work at home or in the real world, whether you are a student or a teacher; you need a good night of sound sleep in order to be at your peak.

The "Think of something good you did today" technique is one of the easiest, most effective ways to settle your mind on positive things in order to get a good night of sleep.

Slow... things ... down.

Sometimes it just seems impossible to take your mind off of stressful things. When something is so stressful in your life that you simply cannot take your mind off of it, what can you do?

Well, what I do when I'm simply can not free my mind of stressful thought is I keep thinking of them. I just think.... really... slow...ly.

Try it right now. It is amazing a how quickly the stress and anxiety levels melt away. If you realize your mind is speeding up.... slow ... it ...back...down-n-n. With just a bit of practice you can have this powerful tool always at the ready.

Relaxing now.

Deep breathing combined with relaxation is a powerful way to go into a deep sleep quickly. As we stress out our body tenses up. Most of the time we really do not realize just how much tension we are carrying around.

I like to go from my toes to the top of my head releasing tension when I'm having trouble getting to sleep. Here's an example to give you an idea of how this works.

I start by laying down in bed on my back. My legs are uncrossed and my hands are by my sides. The room is dark, quiet, and comfortable.

I take a few of my 1-2-3 breaths. Then I say out loud, "Relaxing now" after the next 2 or 3 deep breaths.

I mentally tell myself that I'm going to let myself relax deeply and go into a pleasant, deep sleep. I reassure myself that if anything happens I will become aware of it and instantly awake. If my mind wanders I just bring it back to the relaxation session.

When I feel ready, I begin relaxing my body one area at a time. I say to myself, "Relaxing my feet. Breathing away all the stress and tension". "Letting go." "Letting go now".

And I move from area to area and let the stress melt away. I'm usually sound asleep - or at least greatly relaxed - after this process.

Let go and...

Sometimes overwhelming things happen in life. Things that cause us to have trouble keeping it together. In such circumstances, how do you ever get any sleep?

These are the times, I believe, when you must turn to a higher power.

Mom and I had a saying we used to tell each other, "Let go and let God". We used that saying for more than sleep, of course. I don't want to make this a sermon but sometimes a higher power can give you peace when nothing else can.

Maybe you are just not sleepy.

Sometimes you cannot sleep because you are caught up on your sleep. You are well rested and are not currently requiring sleep. If you feel this is the case, just stay up until you get sleepy. Don't try and force yourself to sleep under this situation.

This rarely happens to me but I do sometimes wake up very early and fully rested. What I do then is simply stay up. I'll try and do something productive and not worry about not sleeping. If I do get sleepy a little later, then I'll go back to bed.

Most people will rarely have trouble falling asleep, once they get on a sleep supporting routine. Still, it is good to have a few standby methods to help you relax into sound sleep when you need them.

Your age, general health, and any chronic conditions can each have an influence on the ease in which you are able to get to sleep. In the next chapter we will take a look at these factors and how they can affect your sleep.

Sleeping Well When You Are a Senior.

Getting older?

Aging affects sleep. Most of us sleep a little less and wake up more as we get older. As long as you feel rested and energetic when you wake up, less sleep is not a problem.

The habits and routines that help younger men and women sleep better work for seniors as well. But in many cases older folks face special conditions and situations that can affect the quality of sleep.

Stresses caused by changes can disrupt sleep. Deaths of people close to you seem to have an even greater effect as the years go by. Changes in a person's physical abilities as they age can cause pain or anxiety. This can make getting proper sleep more difficult.

A huge change in lifestyle for many seniors comes with retirement and planning for the retired lifestyle. Retirement often comes with too much free time and money worries. During the adjustment period, many seniors find it more difficult to sleep well.

A big key to sleeping well is to make it a priority.

At 57 years of age, I guess you could call me a senior citizen. I have been able to sleep well without medications even when going through some very stressful times. I think it is because I follow a sleep strategy and make sleeping well an important priority.

Focusing on getting a good night of sleep only when we go to bed is a weak strategy. Developing good habits throughout the day will help seniors sleep better.

If you have retired recently and have a bundle of free time on your hands, get busy with a hobby or volunteer work. Find something to do that is low stress and fulfilling.

If you find yourself worrying about money, pick up a part time retirement job. A little spending money could settle your nerves and keep you out of the house.

Look at your freed up schedule as giving you the opportunity to reconnect with life passions you had to sacrifice during your work years. Are you a baseball nut? Maybe it's time to help out with a Little League team. Always wanted to write? It's never been easier!

Fill up your idle hours with positives. That will help you doze off at bedtime.

Medical troubles in seniors can make it hard to sleep well.

Even some medications we take to manage our medical conditions can make it more difficult to sleep. Talk to your medical folks. Talk to your doctor and ask your pharmacists. Many times I've found the people behind the counter at the drugstore very helpful.

Sleep disorders.

Conditions such as insomnia, sleep apnea, and restless legs syndrome are more common among the older generation.

The majority of people over age 60 report symptoms of insomnia. It may take them a long time to fall asleep. They may wake up several times during the night. They may wake up early and stay awake. Or they may just wake up feeling tired.

There are many causes of insomnia. Stress due to changes in the person's life can lead to insomnia. Medical conditions can also cause a person to lose sleep. An enlarged prostate can cause men to have to get up to use the bathroom during the night. Urinary incontinence can have the same effect in women.

Any painful condition is going to make it hard for you to get to sleep and to sleep well. Parkinson's and dementia can interfere with a good night's sleep.

Restless legs syndrome is a movement disorder that can make it difficult to fall asleep and stay asleep. While it can occur at any age, it is more frequent in middle aged and older adults. It also can worse as a person ages. Women are about two times more likely than men to have this neurological condition.

The list of medical problems that contribute to insomnia is long.

Habits that interfere with sleeping well at night.

As we age there are several tendencies we develop that make it harder to sleep at night. We take more naps. We exercise less. We do not get outside as much as we used to.

Make sure you have not slipped into any of these bad habits. Reversing these trends is an easy way to improve your chances for a sound night or restful sleep.

Try to limit your naps to 30 minutes or less. Resist the temptation to nap in the evening. Get outside when you can. Take a walk.

As we get older the natural sleep pattern shifts . You may find that you want to go to sleep earlier and get up early as well. Go with it. This is your natural sleep cycle now. Trying to stay up late like you used to will only disrupt your sleep cycle.

Also, as we get older, the body produces less melatonin and a lower level of growth hormone. These lessening levels can cause you to get less deep sleep and sleep can become more fragmented.

Habits you can develop to sleep better.

Exercise regularly.

Aerobic activity , such as walking, will help you sleep. If you exercise vigorously, try to limit exercise to at least 3 hours before bedtime.

Get out in the sun.

A couple of hours in the sun can help regulate your sleep cycle and melatonin levels.

Keep in the dark at night.

You do not want to suppress melatonin production with artificial lights at night. Likewise make sure your bedroom is dark and cool.

Watch the caffeine and alcohol.

They were not any good for you when you were younger. They are even worse now that you've got a few years on you.

Lose some weight.

Do you need to lose a few pounds? Losing excess weight in a healthy way can have the additional benefit of helping you to sleep better.

Medications to help you sleep better.

As we mentioned earlier, sometimes medications can interfere with sleep. But there are medications that can help you sleep better. This is a subject well outside the scope of this book.

Just because you are getting older does not mean you cannot sleep well. If you are hale and hearty without any health issues, you may be able to enjoy nights of sound sleep just by making a few commitments to develop better habits day in and day out.

If you do have health concerns, do not despair. The medical community, including specialist in sleep care can assist you in getting better sleep. Sleep is important for all of us. It is especially vital as we get older.

Getting The Best Sleep When You Are Pregnant.

Sleeping well while pregnant is a chore, so I'm told. If you had bad sleeping habits before becoming pregnant, the sleep disturbances of pregnancy will only make things worse. Leg cramps, snoring, nausea, and heartburn can all interfere with your sleep quality. And a few well timed baby kicks can also wake you up.

So, the first step to sleeping as well as possible during pregnancy is to make sure your basic sleep supporting routine is as in tack as possible. You know the drill. Get up and go to bed on as regular a schedule as possible. Minimize the caffeine. Manage the stress. Get plenty of sunshine. Unwind in the evening. Sleep in a clean, cool, dark room.

But the requirements to sleep well while pregnant go beyond the basics. You'll want to do a few things different and develop some additional supporting habits.

Bland snacks to prevent morning sickness.

It is a good idea to snack on something like crackers before you go to bed. Having food in your stomach can help prevent nausea and minimize morning sickness.

Stick with bland foods and avoid spicy foods entirely. Spicy foods can cause heartburn. Eat a light meal two to three hours before bedtime and finish your day with a light snack.

Go ahead and take a nap and exercise.

Nap for a half hour to a full hour. The rest will help with fatigue and make you more alert. Just do not take that nap too late in the day. An evening nap can make it harder to get to sleep at night.

The same thing goes for exercise. Exercise before the evening hours. Save the time before bed for relaxation.

Become a relaxation ninja.

Brush up on your relaxation methods. There are lots of ways to relax and unwind. Get good at deep breathing techniques. Find a quiet corner in your home and sip on a cup of warm cocoa milk.

Give yourself permission to take a vacation from worry for the night. Think about the good things that happened today.

Take a class.

Classes for pregnant women and their partners can be help relieve anxiety as well as being informative. Classes can teach you about labor and delivery, how to take care of your newborn, and more.

You can meet new friends going through their pregnancies also. Having an empathetic support group is reassuring and will ease your mind. That can only help when the time for sleep rolls around.

Sleep on your left side.

You probably already learned this in class, didn't you? The reason for sleeping on your left side is because this position help blood and nutrients flow to the baby and uterus. It helps you eliminate fluids better as well. Train yourself to sleep on the left side early in your pregnancy.

Large support pillows are also on the market to pregnant women. There are many different styles that wrap around and provide support in key areas. You can also place normal pillows where you need them in order to be more comfortable.

Get comfortable.

If you are having trouble with your breath try propping yourself up while in bed. This helps with heartburn also.

Maternity belts and sleeping bras can provide support as the pregnancy progresses.

Change to a more comfortable mattress. Some pregnant women report relief from egg crate foam or air mattresses. Perhaps one of these would work for you.

In addition to regular pillows and pillows made for pregnancy, there are also pregnancy wedges on the market. These provide another means of support.

Interrupted sleep during pregnancy is normal.

Do not worry if you cannot sleep or wake up during the night. This is to be expected. If you can't sleep just get up. Go to another room and do something relaxing. After a while you will get sleepy. Just go with the flow. Don't add to your worries.

Getting Better Sleep While on Shift Work.

Coping with shift work, especially rotating shift is a big challenge. While some manage better than others, sleeping well while working on the swing shift or graveyard is very difficult. You risk developing a sleep disorder. The best policy is to avoid shift work as much as possible.

But with as many as 1 in 5 workers working shifts, it is often impossible to avoid shift work and keep your job. That being the case, what are the best ways to minimize and counteract the bad effects shift work has on our sleep? Many of the habits that help you sleep soundly under normal conditions are even more important when you work shifts.

Keep a routine.
As much as possible stick with a routine time to go to bed and get up. As long as you are on a set shift try and stick to a consistent schedule.

Avoid caffeine before bedtime and eat healthily.
Set a time several hours before bedtime and stop drinking coffee and any other drinks that have caffeine. A healthy diet is especially important when your normal sleep cycle is out of kilter. Make certain you are getting your nutrition.

Adapt your bedroom for daytime sleep.
Make sure the bedroom is cool and dark. Invest in some blackout shades and a room air conditioner if needed. Make sure your children understand the importance of you getting your sleep.

As much as possible, schedule activities and errands outside or your scheduled sleep hours. It is sometimes tempting to do tasks when you should be sleeping, but realize the importance of your routine.

Exercise.

It is a good idea to plan any exercise or physical activities after you have gotten your sleep. Rev yourself up to go to work and not before you go to bed.

You can nap.

If there is one good thing about shift work it's that you can take naps more liberally. A 30 minute nap just before work or even a quick cat nap during breaks (if allowed) can revive you and keep you sharp. Do not overdo it though. Keep the naps short.

Light therapy.

You can adjust your body's sleep cycle by exposure to bright light. Studies show that artificial bright light can reset your internal clock. clock.

15 to 30 minute sessions with a light box at the right time of day and with the right amount of light intensity can help. There are specialists in light therapy that you can go to in order to develop a plan that works safely.

Minimize the amount of shift work.

I realize this may be unrealistic advice for some. Still, if you are able to get off shift work or minimize the amount of shift work, that is best.

Maybe you can not take as many shifts or transfer to a different department or even get the cushy promotion and live the 9 to 5 life. A more drastic option would be to work somewhere else where shift work in not necessary.

Many times it is just not practical to get off shift work. It may be the best choice for you right now. If so, just realize that you need to take good care of your health. An vital part of good health is sleeping well. It is possible to sleep well in the daytime. But it does take more planning and effort.

Dealing With Jet Lag.

Sleeping in different time zones from one night to the next can wreak havoc on a sleep schedule. Jet lag is a condition that disrupts the body's normal rhythms. Crossing several times zones in an airliner can make you extremely tired and unsettled.

How jet lag affects sleep.
If you have flow east to west for a great distance you know that strange, "What? Is it only 2 P.M. ??" feeling. The natural 24 hour body cycle takes a while to adjust to the new time. For a day or two you'll be adjusting to the sun rising and setting a few hours later than you expect.

East to west.
My policy was to always try to split the difference on the first night, if possible. On a three hour time difference, I'd try and go to bed about an hour and a half earlier on the local time. That would actually be an hour and a half late in my normal time zone.

The farther you travel horizontally, the more nights you'll need to allow for adjustments.

Start adjusting your sleep schedule before the day of the flight.
One trick many veteran travelers use is to start adjusting the sleep cycle in increments a couple of days before hand. Start staying up later and getting up later. A couple of 30 minute adjustments in the days before you leave can help lessen the amount of adjustment you'll need out west.

Nap.
It's ideal if you are comfortable enough to nap on the plane. Just do not overdo the nap. Short naps are helpful. Long naps can make your groggy and lethargic. Bring along earplugs and a sleep mask.

Upon arrival.
There are several helpful things you can do after you've made it to your destination. Seek out the sun and get an ample amount of sunlight.

Eat light. Too much food can make you sleepy. That's not good. You want to stay up until your new bedtime.

You'll be sleeping in a bed that's not your own in a new environment. This can be unsettling and stressful. It's is helpful to bring along some comfort items from home. A picture of your family, a favorite coffee mug, even a pillow, or anything familiar that can be reassuring when you are away from home.

Going from west to east is different.
Heading east the day gets shorter. You're revved up when everyone else is winding down. Some of the some guidelines apply and some are just the opposite.

You can start adjusting your schedule beforehand.
Getting up earlier and going to bed earlier a day or so before you fly east eases the adjustment. I like to get up a hour or so earlier on the flight day. I'm anxious to fly home so it's not a problem.

Do not nap.
Since your day will be missing some time a nap would only make you more awake.

Skip the caffeine.
Maybe a cup of Joe early in the morning but you will want to establish an early cutoff point.

Exercise before you go.
Something aerobic will energize you and take away some pre-flight anxiety.

When you land.

Try to get into your evening relaxation routine as soon as possible. You may need to stay up a little later than usual for the first night. Give yourself a day or so to make the adjustment.

Sleeping soundly during your trip.

You may have to adjust to all sorts of changes at your destination. Changes in temperature, altitude, and humidity can be large. I once left sunny Orlando in March only to land at Chicago O'Hare and 13 inches of snow. Going south to north or vice versa can also present challenges.

Besides the environmental differences, the bedroom environment is probably not going to match the bedroom you created back home. You may have to deal with busy highways just outside your room and loud revelers above, below, or just outside your room.

Use as many of your normal relaxation methods as possible. Cut down sound and light as much as you can. You might even pack a white noise machine or play one of the long running videos of rain or waves crashing that are online.

Adjust your mindset and expect some disturbances in your sleep. Try to go with the flow and do not let things outside of your control escalate. Yes, this may be the worst trip ever. Just realize it is only temporary and really appreciate the comforts of home. You'll be back soon.

Helping Baby Sleep Better.

If your newborn baby sleeps 16 hours a day, then how come you never get any rest? True babies sleep a lot but they get up a lot too. They go from sleep to being awake frequently throughout the day and night in their first three months after being born.

Gradually, the newborn sleeps for a longer period at one time. After the first three months or so, baby should be sleeping for at least a 5 hour stretch during the night with naps during the day. During the first year, the baby should start sleeping for about 10 hours at night. Exactly when he or she will start sleeping longer depends. Each baby is unique.

Helping your baby sleep better at night.

You can encourage a good night's sleep for your baby by actively engaging the infant during waking hours. Keep baby stimulated with play, singing, and movement. Wear them out!

Just like you, your baby needs a soothing routine before sleepy time. Bathing and singing a lullaby can help your little one relax and signal that it is time to rest. Don't play games or do anything to excite the child.

Once the baby is almost ready to go to sleep, put him or her in the crib on the back. Resting on the back helps prevent SIDS (sudden infant death syndrome). The room in which the crib is in should be quiet and dark. Consider placing the baby's crib in your bedroom.

A pacifier can help settle your baby down at night. It also reduces the chances of SIDS. The baby will often stir during the night. Wait a few minutes and see if he goes back to sleep.

When you do care for your baby during the night use a calm soothing voice and keep the lights down low.

It takes time to learn your baby's habits and ways. As a parent, you need to keep a realistic attitude about your baby's sleep schedule and habits.

Each baby has a unique temperament that takes a while to learn. Be flexible and willing to adjust your approach to getting your baby to sleep.

You cannot force your baby into sleep. The goal is to over time help your baby learn that sleep is a pleasant and secure state. Helping your baby see sleep in this light can prevent many sleep disorders as they become older.

Helping your baby stay asleep

Once your baby is sleeping, how do you keep her sleeping?

Keep the bedroom quiet.

Some babies are awaken easily by sudden noises. Some sleep right through much noise. If you have an easily awakened baby, make sure the bedroom is a quiet zone.

Keep the bedroom dark.

Some babies wake up with the first rays of sunlight. Shades that block out the sun rays may help your little one sleep longer.

A cool room but warm sheets.

While a cool room temperature of about 70 degrees is ideal, your baby will prefer not to lay down on cool sheets. Use sheets you have warmed with a warm towel or flannel sheets.

Remove any irritating items from the sleep environment.

Cotton sleepwear instead of synthetic clothing helps some babies to sleep without irritation. Other irritants include pet dander, fumes, cigarette smoke, and hairspray. Airborne irritants that keep your baby awake can come from the most unsuspected sources. Stuffed toys, pillows, blankets, and even the baby canopy.

A little bit of cereal? Clean diapers and more.

A full but not stuffed tummy can help some babies sleep better. Change your babies diaper after a bowel movement. Unless you a treating diaper rash, you can let your baby sleep through a wet diaper. Make sure your baby's nasal passages are clear before bedtime.

Seek help and share responsibilities.
You don't have to go it alone. Baby doctors and grandparents are wonderful resources you can lean on.

Dads can participate, too! It's important for baby and mommy for daddy to take on his share of the nightly duties. Baby needs to get used to being in her father's arms and his unique ways of comforting.

www.ingramcontent.com/pod-product-compliance
Lightning Source LLC
Chambersburg PA
CBHW070819290526
45795CB00002B/761